Copyright © 20

All rights reserved. No part of this publication maybe reproduced, distributed, or transmitted in any form or by any means, including photocopying, recording, or other electronic or mechanical methods, without the prior written permission of the publisher, except in the case of brief quotations embodied in critical reviews and certain other noncommercial uses permitted by copyright law.

Contents

What is neutropenia? 6

Types of neutropenia 6

    Congenital 6

    Cyclic 7

    Autoimmune 7

    Idiopathic 8

What are the symptoms of neutropenia? 8

What causes neutropenia? 10

Who is at risk? 12

Diagnosing neutropenia 12

Treating neutropenia 14

Can you prevent neutropenia? 15

What Is Neutropenic Diet? 17

Who Needs to Follow a Neutropenic Diet? 18

Food Safety Guidelines 20

Foods to eat 21

Foods to avoid 22

Food Storage and Preparation 24

Other Dietary Challenges 27

Preventive Tips 29

Are there medications to avoid while on the neutropenic diet? 31

How does the neutropenic diet help people with cancer? 32

Sample meal plan 32

NEUTROPENIC DIET RECIPES 35

Roasted Cauliflower Salad with Lemon and Capers 35

Vegan Sopa Verde With Parsnips 39

Chicken Meatloaf 42

Mushroom Farrotto 47

Mushroom Farrotto 52

Cumin & Cilantro Marinated Turkey Breast 57

Stir-Fried Celery with Pistachios 59

Veggie Fried Rice 62

Spaghetti with Sausage & Spring Vegetables .. 67

Stuffed Mushrooms 71

Asparagus & Pine Nut Pasta 73

Kale & Ricotta Stuffed Shells 77

Moroccan Spiced Lentil Soup 81

Frittata with Leafy Greens 84

Chicken & Noodles in Coconut Lime Broth 88

Kale and Wild Rice Casserole 92

Baked Mac & Cheese 98

Fall Harvest Salad 102

Strawberry Jello Poke Cake 105

Chipotle Tomatillo Green-Chili Salsa 108

Cheesy Spinach Artichoke Dip 110

Chai Poh Neng 113

What is neutropenia?

Neutropenia is a blood condition characterized by low levels of neutrophils, which are white blood cells that protect your body from infections.

Without enough neutrophils, your body can't fight off bacteria. Having neutropenia increases your risk for many types of infection.

Types of neutropenia

There are four types of neutropenia:

Congenital

Congenital neutropenia is present at birth. Severe congenital neutropenia is also called Kostmann syndrome. It causes very low neutrophil levels and in some cases, complete lack of neutrophils. This puts infants and young children at risk for serious infections.

Cyclic

Cyclic neutropenia is present at birth and causes neutrophil counts to vary in a 21-day cycle. A period of neutropenia may last a few days, followed by normal levels for the rest of the cycle. The cycle then begins again.

Autoimmune

With autoimmune neutropenia, your body makes antibodies that fight your neutrophils. These antibodies kill the neutrophils, causing neutropenia.

Autoimmune neutropenia is most common in infants and young children, with the average age of diagnosis between 7 and 9 monthsTrusted Source.

Idiopathic

Idiopathic neutropenia develops any time in life and can affect anyone. The cause is unknown.

What are the symptoms of neutropenia?

Neutropenia symptoms can range from mild to severe. The lower the level of neutrophils, the more intense the symptoms.

Typical symptoms include:

- fever

- pneumonia

- sinus infections

- otitis media (ear infection)

- gingivitis (gum inflammation)

- omphalitis (navel infection)

- skin abscesses

Severe congenital neutropenia can have serious symptoms. The symptoms often include bacterial infections. These infections can grow on the skin and in the digestive and respiratory systems.

The symptoms of cyclic neutropenia recur in 3-week cycles. Infections can increase when neutrophil levels fall.

The symptoms of autoimmune and idiopathic neutropenia include infections. They're usually not as severe as those in congenital forms.

What causes neutropenia?

Neutropenia can be triggered by:

- chemotherapy

- radiation therapy

- the use of certain drugs

Other causes include:

- Shwachman-Diamond syndrome, which is an inherited condition affecting many organs and often characterized by bone marrow and pancreatic failure

- glycogen-storage disease type 1b, which is a rare inherited disorder that affects blood sugar levels

- leukemia

- viral illnesses

- severe aplastic anemia

- Fanconi anemia

- conditions that affect bone marrow

- infections, both viral and bacterial, including HIV, hepatitis, tuberculosis, and Lyme disease

- deficiencies in certain vitamins and minerals, including B12, folic acid, and copper

According to the U.S. National Library of Medicine, most people with severe congenital neutropenia have no family history of the condition.

Who is at risk?

The risk of neutropenia is increased by certain conditions, such as:

- cancer

- leukemia

- a weakened immune system

Chemotherapy and radiation therapy also raise the risk.

Idiopathic neutropenia affects people of all ages, but people over 70 are at higher risk. Men and women are at equal risk.

Diagnosing neutropenia

Your doctor can use these tests to diagnose neutropenia:

- Complete blood count (CBC). This test measures neutrophil counts. Intermittent CBC tests can help your doctor check for changes in neutrophil count three times per week for 6 weeks.

- Antibody blood test. This test checks for autoimmune neutropenia.

- Bone marrow aspirate. This procedure tests bone marrow cells.

- Bone marrow biopsy. This involves testing a piece of the bony part of bone marrow.

- Cytogenetic and molecular testing. This testing helps your healthcare provider study the structures of the cells.

Treating neutropenia

Most cases of neutropenia can be treated with granulocyte-colony stimulating factors (G-CSF). This is a synthetic copy of the hormone that causes neutrophils to grow in the bone marrow. G-CSF can increase the number of neutrophils.

G-CSF is usually given as a daily subcutaneous (under the skin) injection. The treatment sometimes includes bone marrow transplants. This is usually when leukemia is present or G-CSF doesn't work.

The following therapies can also treat infections that occur due to the disorder:

- antibiotics

- anti-inflammatory drugs

- corticosteroids
- cytokines
- glucocorticoids
- immunoglobulins
- immunosuppressive drugs
- white blood cell transfusions
- vitamins

Can you prevent neutropenia?

No specific prevention for neutropenia is known. However, the National Neutropenia Network advises the following to reduce complications:

- Maintain good oral hygiene. Get regular dental exams, and use an antibacterial mouthwash.
- Keep vaccinations current.

- Get medical care for a fever above 101.3°F (38.5°C).

- Wash your hands thoroughly.

- Care for cuts and scrapes.

- Use antibiotics and antifungals as directed.

- Know how to reach your doctor and hospital.

- Talk with your doctor before traveling out of the country.

These preventive lifestyle measures can help you to reduce potential complications of neutropenia. Talk with your doctor about any symptoms that arise, and always know how to reach your doctor and hospital.

What Is Neutropenic Diet?

The neutropenic diet is the term used to describe food handling and selection practices that reduce the risk of bacterial infection from foods. Also known as the antimicrobial diet, it is typically used to prevent foodborne infections in people with severely weakened immune systems, such as those undergoing chemotherapy.

The diet is named after the defensive white blood cells, called neutrophils, that are the first responders to infection. Safe food handling, as well as the avoidance of certain foods, is believed to reduce the risk of infection in people with suppressed immune system.

Although a number of researchers believe that the restrictive nature of the neutropenic diet can lead to malnutrition,1 safe food handling is considered imperative to lowering the risk of chemotherapy-induced neutropenia. Whether the neutropenic diet is effective in preventing infection a subject of ongoing debate.

Who Needs to Follow a Neutropenic Diet?

Doctors often recommend this diet before and after certain types of chemotherapy and other cancer treatments. A blood test called an absolute neutrophil count (ANC) can help determine the body's ability to fight off infection. Many cancer patients have this blood test done routinely. When the ANC is less than 500 cells/mm3, the patient is often instructed to follow a neutropenic diet. This diet should be followed until the doctor tells the patient to resume his or her regular diet.

Patients undergoing autologous stem cell transplants typically follow this diet during the pre-transplant chemotherapy and for the first 3 or more months after transplant. Patients undergoing allogeneic stem cell transplants typically follow this diet during the pre-transplant chemotherapy and continue on it until they no longer take immunosuppressive drugs. The transplant team will tell the patient how long to follow this diet.

People who have had an organ transplant or who are being treated for HIV/AIDS also may need to follow this diet. If you are not sure if you should follow this diet, check with your doctor, nurse, or dietitian.

Food Safety Guidelines

The prevention of bacterial transmission is the primary aim of the neutropenic diet. Oncologists insist that handwashing is the first-line defense against infection and the one that most people forgot. Food safety guidelines include:

• Wash your hands frequently, before and after eating.

• Avoid raw meats and eggs. Be sure to cook all the way.

• Wash raw fruits and vegetables.

• Avoid sharing food even with loved ones.

• Do not share personal eating utensils.

- Keep surfaces clean in the kitchen and dining room.

Foods to eat

Foods you're allowed to eat on the neutropenic diet include:

- Dairy: all pasteurized milk and dairy products, such as cheese, yogurt, ice cream, and sour cream

- Starches: all breads, cooked pastas, chips, French toast, pancakes, cereal, cooked sweet potatoes, beans, corn, peas, whole grains, and fries

- Vegetables: all cooked or frozen vegetables

- Fruits: all canned and frozen fruit and fruit juices, along with thoroughly washed and peeled thick-skinned fruits like bananas, oranges, and grapefruit

- Protein: thoroughly cooked (well-done) meats and canned meats, as well as hard-cooked or boiled eggs and pasteurized egg substitutes

- Beverages: all tap, bottled, or distilled water, as well as canned or bottled drinks, individually canned sodas, and instant or brewed tea and coffee

Foods to avoid

Foods you should eliminate while following the neutropenic diet include:

- Dairy: unpasteurized milk and yogurt, yogurt made with live or active cultures, soft cheeses (Brie, feta, sharp Cheddar), cheeses with mold

(Gorgonzola, blue cheese), aged cheeses, cheeses with uncooked vegetables, and Mexican-style cheeses like queso

- Raw starches: bread with raw nuts, uncooked pasta, raw oats, and raw grains

- Vegetables: raw vegetables, salads, uncooked herbs and spices, and fresh sauerkraut

- Fruits: unwashed raw fruits, unpasteurized fruit juices, and dried fruits

- Protein: raw or undercooked meat, deli meats, sushi, cold meat, and undercooked eggs with runny yolk

- Beverages: sun tea, cold brewed tea, eggnog made with raw eggs, fresh apple cider, and homemade lemonade

Food Storage and Preparation

Bacterial contamination will often occur during the preparation and storage of food. Recommendations for food preparation and storage include:

• Keep hot foods hot (over 140° F)

• Keep cold foods cold (under 40° F).

• Eat defrosted foods right away. Do not refreeze.

• Refrigerate foods at or below 40° F.

• Do not thaw meat, seafood, or chicken at room temperature. Use the microwave or refrigerator instead.

- After buying perishable foods, eat them within two hours.

- Eggs, cream, and mayonnaise-based foods should not be kept outside of the refrigerator for more than an hour.

- Wash fruits and vegetables thoroughly with water before cutting or peeling. Wash lettuce leaves one at a time.

- Do not use chemical-based rinses.

- Rinse "prewashed" salads.

- Avoid raw vegetable sprouts.

- Toss food that smells funny or shows signs of spoilage.

- Avoid pre-cut fruits and vegetables.

- Wash the tops of canned foods with soap and water before opening.

- Use a different utensil for eating and tasting foods while cooking.

- Throw away eggs with cracked shells.

- Do not use the same cutting board or utensil for meat preparation as for vegetable and fruit preparation.

- Use a meat thermometer to make sure meats are cooked to the proper temperature.

Some oncologists use the mnemonic "PICKY" to help people remember safe food practices. The letters in "PICKY" stand for:

- Practice handwashing.

- Inspect foods before you cook them.

- Clean and scrub fruits and vegetables.

- Keep all cooking surfaces clean.

- Yucky, moldy food should be thrown away.

Other Dietary Challenges

In addition to safe food handling, people going through chemotherapy often have other challenges as well. Some of these include:

- Mouth sores: Painful sores in the mouth are common, but choosing foods that are less likely to irritate the mouth can do wonders. Avoiding citrus foods, sharp foods (such as toast), and more is often advised.

- Taste changes: Some chemotherapy drugs can make everything you eat taste metallic and has been coined metal mouth. Choosing foods with strong flavors and eating with plastic utensils can be helpful, among other changes.

- Nausea and vomiting: Nausea and vomiting certainly interfere with eating, but there are now many options to control these symptoms. Talk to your oncologist.

- Loss of appetite: Even if you simply don't feel like eating, there are tips that can help you get adequate nutrition.

- Cancer fatigue: Fatigue is one of the most annoying symptoms of cancer treatment, and is not uncommonly the reason why people don't eat as healthily as they should. Make sure to ask for help with cooking, shopping, and cleaning up. Stock your pantry with easy-to-prepare foods such as canned soups, frozen entrees, frozen vegetables, and packaged puddings.

If you are concerned about food handling or foods to eat while on chemotherapy, talk to your oncologist and ask if seeing an oncology nutritionist might be helpful.

Preventive Tips

In addition to safe food practices, there are many ways in which you can reduce your risk of developing an infection during chemotherapy, especially when your white blood cell count is low.

While we often think about avoiding people who have a cough or runny nose, our pets can also be a source of infection. Birds, turtles, and reptiles such as lizards and snakes can carry the bacteria Salmonella, which can be life-threatening in people with severely suppressed immune systems.4

Cat litter boxes are a common source of a protozoan infection called toxoplasmosis.5 During chemotherapy, you should assign the task of cleaning the litter box to a family member or friend.

When your immune system is suppressed, you would do best to avoid crowds or enclosed spaces such as an airplane, especially during cold and flu season.

Are there medications to avoid while on the neutropenic diet?

Don't take supplements, homeopathic remedies, or herbal products (such as St.-John's wort or traditional Chinese medicines) unless you've discussed it with your cancer care team. Because there are no federal standards for these products in the United States, the way they're processed and stored may pose health risks. Microbes in these items can also cause an infection. In addition, the products themselves could interfere with or change the activity of a prescription medication.

How does the neutropenic diet help people with cancer?

Following a neutropenic diet can help prevent foodborne illness in someone with a weakened immune system. People with cancer may have a weakened immune system due to the disease. Chemotherapy, radiation therapy, and a stem cell transplant can also cause a weakened immune system.

Sample meal plan

Breakfast

1- large egg scrambled

Medium biscuit with 1tsp butter and 1 tsp Jelly

1/2 cup apple juice

1/2 cup 2% milk

Coffee or tea

Morning snack

1cup dry cereal

1 cup 2% milk

2 Tbsp dried fruit

Lunch

Baked Meat loaf/ gravy

1/2 cooked corn

1/2 cup canned peaches

Slice wheat bread

Butter or margarine

Coffee or tea

1 cup 2% milk

Afternoon snack

1 cup of milkshake or high protein drink

Dinner

3 ounces Baked or Roasted Chicken

1/2 cup oven fried potatoes

1/2 cup glazed carrots

Dinner roll with butter or margarine

1/2 cup fruit cocktail

Coffee or tea

Evening Snack

Slice pound cake with whip topping

NEUTROPENIC DIET RECIPES

Trying neutropenic-friendly recipes is a great way to explore new flavors and find new favorite dishes while looking after your health. In this part are nourishing abs diet recipes for you to enjoy.

Roasted Cauliflower Salad with Lemon and Capers

Prepartion time

5 minutes

Ingredients

- 1 medium to large cauliflower
- 1 cup water

- 1 1/2 tablespoons olive oil

Lemon Caper Dressing

- ¼ cup olive oil
- 1½ tablespoons fresh lemon juice
- 2 tablespoons water
- ¼ cup salted capers, rinsed well
- salt to taste

Instructions

1. Pre-heat the oven to 425F.
2. Break the cauliflower into large florets.

3. Place in a single layer in a sauté pan and add 1 cup of the water.

4. Sprinkle with salt.

5. Cover and bring to a boil over a medium high flame.

6. Steam for 5 minutes or until the florets can just be pierced with a fork. Drain.

7. Set the florets aside on paper towel to absorb any excess moisture.

8. Break the largest florets into 2-3 pieces (this can be done ahead of time).

9. Line a baking sheet with parchment paper and drizzle with 1 ½ tablespoons of the olive oil.

10. Place the drained cauliflower onto the prepared baking sheet in a single layer. Turn the florets to coat in the olive oil.

11. Roast in the oven for 10 minutes.

12. Turn the florets over and cook 10 minutes more to brown the other sides. The florets will be soft and covered in brown spots.

13. Meanwhile make the dressing.

14. Put the lemon juice in a large bowl.

15. Gradually beat in the remaining olive oil.

16. If the dressing seems too sharp, beat in the water a teaspoon at a time until desired sharpness is reached.

17. Stir in the capers. Let sit for 5 minutes. Taste for salt.

18. Add the roasted cauliflower and toss to coat.

19. Let sit for 10 minutes for the flavors to blend.

20. Serve at room temperature.

Vegan Sopa Verde With Parsnips

Prepartion time

20 minutes

Ingredients

- 2 tablespoons olive oil

- 1 cup parsnips, large diced

- ½ cup onion, large diced

- 3 garlic cloves, chopped

- 2 sprigs thyme
- 1 teaspoons cumin
- 2 tablespoons smoked paprika
- 8 cups water or stock
- 4 cups thinly sliced kale
- ½ cup lemon juice
- salt to taste

Instructions

1. In a medium pot over medium heat, add olive oil.

2. Once warm add parsnips and onions.

3. Sprinkle with a little salt and cook until onions are translucent, about 5 minutes.

4. Add garlic, thyme, cumin, and smoked paprika to pot.

5. Season with salt and sauté for about 2 minutes, until garlic is fragrant.

6. Add the water or stock.

7. Bring to a boil over a high heat.

8. Lower the heat to medium.

9. Cook until parsnips are fully cooked and fork tender, about 30 minutes.

10. Allow soup to cool slightly.

11. Transfer soup to a blender in batches.

12. Blend each batch until smooth before starting the next.

13. Pour blended soup back into the pot.

14. When all is blended bring to a simmer over a medium flame.

15. Add kale and cook just until kale is wilted and bright green, about 5 minutes.

16. Finish with lemon juice and serve.

Chicken Meatloaf

Prepartion time

20 minutes

Ingredients

- 1 tablespoon olive oil
- 1 sprig fresh thyme, leaves stripped
- ½ an onion, finely diced
- 2 carrots, finely diced
- 1 small leek or 2 scallions, finely diced
- 1 clove garlic, finely chopped
- 2 tablespoons chopped parsley
- 1 tomato, finely diced (optional)
- 1 large egg, beaten
- ⅓ cup Worcestershire sauce
- 1 teaspoon Thai chili sauce to taste (optional)
- Salt and pepper, to taste
- 1 pound ground chicken

- 1 cup whole wheat breadcrumbs, soaked in a little milk or stock

- 1 cup marinara sauce (or 1/4 cup Quick Tomato Sauce), heated through

Instructions

1. Preheat the oven to 375 degrees.

2. Lightly butter a small gratin dish or loaf tin, set aside.

3. Heat the oil over a medium-high heat.

4. When it is hot, add the thyme, onion, carrots and leeks and cook, stirring, until they start to soften.

5. Turn the heat down to medium-low, cover and sweat the vegetables for until they are soft, about 10 minutes.

6. Do not let them burn!

7. Add the garlic and parsley, turn the heat back up and sauté for a couple of minutes.

8. Add the chopped tomato, if using.

9. Cook for another 5 minutes, turn off heat and set aside.

10. Beat the egg, 2½ tablespoons of the Worcestershire sauce and the Thai chili sauce together.

11. Add salt and pepper.

12. In a large bowl combine ground chicken with the vegetables and mix with a spatula.

13. Add the beaten egg mixture and combine.

14. Gradually add in the breadcrumbs and mix well.

15. Turn the mixture into the gratin dish and smooth the top.

16. Bake in the middle of the oven for 20 minutes, then gently spread a tablespoon of tomato sauce over the top of the meatloaf and sprinkle the rest of Worcester sauce over it.

17. Return to the oven and finish cooking for 15 to 20 minutes. The loaf should be well browned, firm to the touch and drawn away slightly from the sides of the dish.

18. Serve with the remaining tomato sauce and either mashed potatoes or pasta, such as macaroni or orzo.

Mushroom Farrotto

Prepartion time

30 minutes

Ingredients

- 2 ounces dried shiitake mushrooms soaked in 3 cups of boiling water

- 3 tablespoons extra virgin olive oil, divided

- 1 onion, diced

- 1 stalk celery, diced

- 1 carrot, diced

- 2 cups farro, rinsed, soaked overnight and drained

- 1 lemon, juiced and mixed with 1/3 cup water

- 1 cup water or vegetable stock as needed

- 2 cloves garlic, thinly sliced

- 2 shallots, thinly sliced

- ½ teaspoon dried Thyme or 1 large sprig of fresh

- 1 lb Baby Bella or Portabella mushrooms, cut into ¼ " slices

- ¼ cup freshly grated Parmesan cheese (optional)

- 2 tablespoons chopped Italian flat leaf parsley

Instructions

1. Soak the dried shitake mushrooms for 30 minutes while you prep the vegetables.

2. Drain, reserving the soak water.

3. Take the soaked mushrooms, discard the woody stems and roughly chop. Set aside.

4. Strain the soak water through a fine sieve. Set aside.

5. Heat 1 tablespoon of the olive oil in a Dutch oven over a medium high flame.

6. When it shimmers, add the onion, celery, and carrot.

7. Sprinkle with salt and cook stirring until the onion is transparent and the vegetables have softened, about 5 minutes.

8. Add the drained farro. Cook until the juices in the pan are absorbed.

9. Add lemon-water mixture and mushroom soaking water, and cook until the farro is 'al dente' - tender but still a little chewy – and the water absorbed, about 30 minutes. If the farro is dry but still underdone, add the additional water or stock, a ¼ cup at a time.

10. Meanwhile, in a sauté pan heat the remaining olive oil over a medium high flame.

11. Add the garlic, shallots and dried thyme. Sauté until the shallots start to color, about 3 minutes.

12. Add the chopped dried mushrooms, cook 1-2 minutes then add the sliced Portabella mushrooms.

13. Sprinkle with salt and cook until they wilt, about 5-8 minutes.

14. Add the white wine and reduce until it starts to look syrupy.

15. Cover the pan and turn off the heat.

16. Let the mushrooms sit for 5-10 minutes or until the farro is cooked.

17. Stir in the sautéed mushrooms and all their juices into the cooked farro.

18. Stir the grated cheese if using. Taste for salt.

19. Garnish with chopped parsley and serve immediately.

Mushroom Farrotto

Prepartion time

30 minutes

Ingredients

- 2 ounces dried shiitake mushrooms soaked in 3 cups of boiling water

- 3 tablespoons extra virgin olive oil, divided

- 1 onion, diced

- 1 stalk celery, diced

- 1 carrot, diced

- 2 cups farro, rinsed, soaked overnight and drained (See Ann's Tips)

- 1 lemon, juiced and mixed with 1/3 cup water

- 1 cup water or vegetable stock as needed

- 2 cloves garlic, thinly sliced

- 2 shallots, thinly sliced

- ½ teaspoon dried Thyme or 1 large sprig of fresh

- 1 lb Baby Bella or Portabella mushrooms, cut into ¼ " slices

- ¼ cup freshly grated Parmesan cheese (optional)

- 2 tablespoons chopped Italian flat leaf parsley

Instructions

1. Soak the dried shitake mushrooms for 30 minutes while you prep the vegetables. Drain, reserving the soak water.

2. Take the soaked mushrooms, discard the woody stems and roughly chop. Set aside.

3. Strain the soak water through a fine sieve. Set aside.

4. Heat 1 tablespoon of the olive oil in a Dutch oven over a medium high flame.

5. When it shimmers, add the onion, celery, and carrot.

6. Sprinkle with salt and cook stirring until the onion is transparent and the vegetables have softened, about 5 minutes.

7. Add the drained farro.

8. Cook until the juices in the pan are absorbed.

9. Add lemon-water mixture and mushroom soaking water, and cook until the farro is 'al dente' - tender but still a little chewy – and the water absorbed, about 30 minutes. If the farro is dry but still underdone, add the additional water or stock, a ¼ cup at a time.

10. Meanwhile, in a sauté pan heat the remaining olive oil over a medium high flame.

11. Add the garlic, shallots and dried thyme.

12. Sauté until the shallots start to color, about 3 minutes.

13. Add the chopped dried mushrooms, cook 1-2 minutes then add the sliced Portabella mushrooms.

14. Sprinkle with salt and cook until they wilt, about 5-8 minutes.

15. Add the white wine and reduce until it starts to look syrupy.

16. Cover the pan and turn off the heat.

17. Let the mushrooms sit for 5-10 minutes or until the farro is cooked.

18. Stir in the sautéed mushrooms and all their juices into the cooked farro.

19. Stir the grated cheese if using.

20. Taste for salt.

21. Garnish with chopped parsley and serve immediately.

Cumin & Cilantro Marinated Turkey Breast

Prepartion time

20 minutes

Ingredients

- ¼ cup fresh mint leaves
- ¼ cup flat leaf parsley leaves
- ¼ cup cilantro
- 2 garlic cloves, smashed and peeled
- ¼ cup lemon juice
- 1 teaspoon ground cumin
- ½ teaspoon ground white pepper

- 1 (2½-pound) boneless turkey breast

- Salt, to taste

Instructions

1. In a food processor combine the mint leaves, parsley, cilantro, garlic, lemon juice, cumin, and white pepper and process until smooth.

2. Reserve ¼ cup of the marinade in the refrigerator.

3. Pour the rest of marinade into a re-sealable plastic bag.

4. Put the turkey in the bag with the marinade, and seal.

5. Massage the marinade into the meat, and place on a plate to catch any leaks.

6. Leave in the refrigerator for at least 4 hours, preferably overnight.

7. Preheat the oven to 400 degrees.

8. Remove the turkey from the marinade and place on a baking sheet.

9. Roast the turkey for 20 minutes then pour the reserved marinade over the turkey, turn down the heat to 350 and cook for another 30 minutes, or until the turkey is done.

10. Let rest for 10 minutes before slicing or serving.

Stir-Fried Celery with Pistachios

Prepartion time

10 minutes

Ingredients

- 1 tablespoon peanut oil

- 2 cloves of garlic, sliced

- 1 large shallot, diced

- 6-8 sticks of celery

- 1/4 cup shelled, unsalted, pistachios

- 1/4 cup water divided

- 2 tablespoons Chinese seasoning sauce (see Ann's Tips)

- 1 cup sunflower sprouts

- salt

Instructions

1. Heat the peanut oil in a wok over a medium high flame.

2. When hot, add the garlic and as soon as it starts to color, about 30 seconds, add the diced shallot.

3. Stir fry until until the shallot starts to color, about 3-5 minutes.

4. Add the celery and the pistachios.

5. Sprinkle with a little salt.

6. Cook stirring until the celery is starting to get tender but is still very crisp, about 2 minutes.

7. Add 2 tablespoons of the water.

8. As soon as it bubbles, add the Chinese seasoning sauce.

9. Cook stirring until the liquid gets syrupy, about 2 minutes. The steam from this will finish cooking the celery.

10. Add the remaining water and bring to a boil.

11. Add the sunflower sprouts.

12. Cook stirring until the sprouts" leaves change color to bright green, but before they begin to wilt, about 30 seconds.

13. Serve immediately with brown rice.

Veggie Fried Rice

Prepartion time

20 minutes

Ingredients

- 2 eggs, lightly beaten
- 1 tablespoon water
- 1 teaspoon plus 3 tablespoons peanut or canola oil (plus an extra 2 teaspoons if needed)
- 2½ tablespoons soy sauce
- 1 teaspoon sugar
- ½ inch ginger root, peeled and finely diced
- 2 medium onions, finely diced
- 1 cup carrots, finely diced
- 1 cup canned sliced water chestnuts

- ¾ teaspoon salt

- 1 teaspoon peanut or canola oil

- 2 to 3 scallions, finely sliced, divided

- 1 (10 ounce) bag of green peas

- 2 cup cooked Brown Rice

- 1 cup bean sprouts

- 2 to 3 large leaves of cabbage, shredded

- 2 tablespoons chopped cilantro (optional or to taste)

Instructions

1. Whisk the eggs, water, and salt together in a small bowl.

2. Heat 2 teaspoons of oil in a skillet over a medium-high heat.

3. Pour the eggs into the pan.

4. Tip the pan from side-to-side to quickly spread the eggs into a thin omelet.

5. When the eggs are just set, slide onto a plate, roll and cut into ¼-inch strips and then across into a dice. Set aside.

6. In a small bowl, mix the sugar and soy sauce and stir until the sugar has dissolved. Set aside.

7. Heat the remaining 3 tablespoons of oil over a medium-high flame in a wok or wide skillet.

8. Add the diced ginger.

9. Let it sizzle for a few minutes then add the onion, carrots, and water chestnuts and stir-fry until they start to soften.

10. While the onions and vegetables are cooking, heat 1 teaspoon oil in a small saucepan.

11. Add half of the scallions, let them sizzle for a second, then add the frozen peas plus 2 teaspoons of water.

12. Cover and cook until the peas are tender. Set aside.

13. Add the diced eggs, and the soy sauce and sugar mixture to the vegetables.

14. Cook stirring until they are well coated.

15. Add the cooked rice and stir to mix.

16. Add the peas and any liquid in their pot.

17. Stir to mix.

18. Cook until the rice has heated through.

19. Add the remaining scallions, the shredded cabbage, bean sprouts, and cilantro. Toss together until well mixed.

20. Once the cabbage has wilted, check for seasoning and serve immediately.

Spaghetti with Sausage & Spring Vegetables

Prepartion time

30 minutes

Ingredients

- 1 pound whole-wheat spaghetti

- 1 tablespoons olive oil

- ½ cup red onion, chopped

- 1 garlic clove, minced

- 3 chicken sausage links, sliced

- 1 yellow squash, julienned

- 1 cup asparagus, cut in 2-inch pieces

- 1 cup fava beans, shelled and peeled

- 1 lemon, juiced

- 1 tablespoon butter

- ½ cup pecorino Romano cheese, shredded

- Salt

- Pepper

Instructions

1. Bring a pot of salted water to a boil.

2. Add pasta to the boiling water and cook until al dente, following package directions minus 1 minute.

3. In a saucepan, heat olive oil on medium heat.

4. Add onion, garlic and chicken sausage to the pan and cook for about 5 minutes until the onions are translucent and the sausage is slightly brown.

5. Add the squash, asparagus, and fava beans to the pan.

6. Add about a ½ cup of pasta cooking water to the pan and cook for about 5 minutes, until the vegetables are soft.

7. Season with lemon juice, salt and pepper.

8. Once the pasta is cooked, drain the water and add it to the pan with the vegetables.

9. Add the butter and cheese to the pan and mix everything to combine.

10. Serve while warm.

Stuffed Mushrooms

Prepartion time

20 minutes

Ingredients

- 2 tablespoons olive oil

- 4 cloves garlic, smashed and thinly sliced

- 2 tablespoons pine nuts

- 4 cups chopped arugula

- 2 tablespoons golden raisins

- Salt, to taste

- 1 cup cooked quinoa

- 6 small portabella tops

Instructions

1. Preheat the oven to 350 degrees. Lightly oil a large baking tray.

2. In a wide sauté pan, heat the olive oil over medium-high heat.

3. Add the garlic and pine nuts, cook just until the garlic is beginning to turn golden, about 3 minutes.

4. Add the arugula, raisins, and salt.

5. Cook for another 3 minutes or until the arugula is well wilted.

6. Turn off the heat and stir in the quinoa.

7. Place the portabella tops, gill side up, in the prepared baking tray and sprinkle with salt and drizzle with olive oil.

8. Evenly divide the quinoa mixture into the mushroom tops, and cover the tray with foil.

9. Bake for 20 minutes, then for 5 minutes uncovered.

10. Serve warm or at room temperature.

Asparagus & Pine Nut Pasta

Prepartion time

30 minutes

Ingredients

- 3 tablespoons pine nuts, lightly toasted

- 1 bunch thin green asparagus (about 1-pound) washed, tough root ends snapped off

- 8 ounces whole wheat penne or rigatoni (2-ounces per person)

- 2 tablespoons olive oil

- 2 cloves garlic, smashed, peeled and thinly sliced

- 1 dried cayenne pepper pod or other dried chili, de-seeded (optional)

- 3 tablespoons chopped flat-leaf Italian parsley

- 1 tablespoon freshly grated Parmesan cheese

- Salt and black pepper, to taste

Instructions

1. In a large stockpot boil enough water for pasta.

2. Add 1 tablespoon of salt.

3. Cut the asparagus roughly the same length as the pasta you"re using.

4. When the pasta water comes to a boil, add the salt and bring it back to a rolling boil, then add the pasta.

5. Cook for 6 minutes.

6. Add the asparagus to the boiling pasta and cook together for 2 minutes.

7. Drain, reserving 1½ cup of the pasta water.

8. Both the pasta and the asparagus should be very al dente.

9. While the pasta is cooking, heat the olive oil over medium-high heat in a wide, deep skillet or wok.

10. When the oil is hot, add the garlic and the chili pepper and stir-fry until the garlic is golden, about 5 minutes.

11. Lower the heat if the garlic is turning brown too quickly.

12. Add the parsley and cook for 1 minute.

13. Add a ¼ cup of the reserved pasta water to the pan and bring to a simmer.

14. Add the pine nuts.

15. Turn down heat to medium, adding more pasta water if the pan gets too dry.

16. Mix in the pasta and asparagus.

17. Add the grated cheese and half of the remaining reserved water.

18. Turn up the heat and bring back to a boil.

19. Cook stirring for 1 minute.

20. Add more water, 1/4 cup at a time, if the pasta looks too dry, it should be slightly saucy.

21. Taste for salt then serve with a grind of black pepper.

Kale & Ricotta Stuffed Shells

Prepartion time

20 minutes

Ingredients

- 1 pound kale leaves, washed and stems removed

- 2 garlic cloves, peeled

- Salt, to taste

- 12 ounces whole wheat jumbo pasta shells (see Ann's Tips)

- 2 teaspoons olive oil

- 10-ounces (1¼ cup) ricotta cheese

- 1 cup basil leaves packed

- 1 large egg

- ½ cup grated Parmesan cheese, 2 tablespoons reserved for topping

- 4 cups Quick Tomato Sauce

- 1 cup grated mozzarella cheese

Instructions

1. Preheat the oven to 350 degrees. Lightly oil a 9- by 12-inch baking tray.

2. Fill a medium bowl halfway with cold water and ice. Set aside.

3. Bring a large pot of salted water to boil.

4. Drop in the kale leaves and garlic cloves and boil for 2 minutes.

5. Using a slotted spoon, remove the kale leaves and garlic cloves and drop them into the prepared ice water.

6. Bring the same pot of water to boil and add in the pasta. Cook for 2 to 3 minutes less than package instructions.

7. Drain the pasta and toss with 2 teaspoons of olive oil.

8. Meanwhile, drain the kale and squeeze out the excess water.

9. Coarsely chop, then blend the chopped kale with the garlic cloves, ricotta, salt, basil leaves, egg, and Parmesan cheese.

10. Fill the pasta shells with a scant 1 tablespoon of the kale ricotta mixture and place in the prepared baking pan.

11. Top the stuffed shells with the Quick Tomato Sauce and sprinkle with the mozzarella cheese and the reserved Parmesan.

12. Cover with foil and bake for 20 minutes, then uncover and bake for another 10 minutes, or until the cheese is turning golden brown.

13. Serve hot.

Moroccan Spiced Lentil Soup

Prepartion time

20 minutes

Ingredients

- 1 tablespoon olive oil

- 1 medium onion, diced

- 1 medium carrot, diced

- 1 celery stalk, diced

- 1 bay leaf

- 2 garlic cloves, minced

- ½ teaspoon turmeric
- ½ stick of cinnamon
- ½ teaspoon ground ginger
- 2 tablespoons tomato paste
- ¾ cup canned chopped tomatoes
- Salt, to taste
- 1 cup large green lentils
- 20 sprigs cilantro, tied together with kitchen twine
- 4 cups water
- 1 tablespoon red wine vinegar or lemon juice (optional)

Instructions

1. In a stockpot, heat the olive over medium heat.

2. Add the onion, carrot, celery and bay leaf.

3. Cook for 8 minutes, or until the onion is translucent.

4. Add the garlic, turmeric, cinnamon stick, and ground ginger.

5. Cook, stirring for 2 minutes.

6. Add the tomato paste, chopped tomato, and salt.

7. Cook for 5 minutes, stirring occasionally, or until the tomatoes have turned orangey.

8. Add the lentils, cilantro sprigs and 4 cups of water.

9. Bring to a boil, then simmer for 30 minutes, or until the lentils are very soft.

10. Add more water if the soup is too thick.

11. Remove the cilantro sprigs, stir in vinegar or lemon juice, cook for 1 minute then serve.

Frittata with Leafy Greens

Prepartion time

20 minutes

Ingredients

- 1 bunch leafy greens (spinach, chard, kale, dandelion, or collard)
- 3 eggs

- 2 tablespoons chopped chives (garlic chives give extra flavor if you can find them)
- 2 tablespoons olive oil
- 2 large shallots, peeled, chopped and sliced
- 3 tablespoons chopped Italian parsley
- Salt and pepper

Instructions

1. Strip the tender greens from any tough stalks. If using chard, dice and reserve the stems. Wash the greens well.

2. Place in a large pan with the water that clings to their leaves.

3. Sprinkle with a little salt.

4. Steam until the leaves have wilted down and are tender.

5. Drain and squeeze out any excess moisture.

6. Coarsely chop and set aside.

7. Beat the eggs in a bowl with salt, pepper and 1 tablespoon of water.

8. Stir in the chopped chives, if using. Set aside.

9. In a large frying pan, slowly sauté the shallots in oil until they are caramelized and a rich gold color, 5-8 minutes over a medium-low heat.

10. Raise the heat to medium-high and add the cooked greens to the shallots.

11. Sauté for 2 minutes.

12. Add the parsley and sauté to mix.

13. Tip the greens into the egg mixture and mix well, then pour everything back into the frying pan.

14. Smooth with a spatula to form a thin, crepe-like frittata.

15. Cook until the frittata is half set and browned where it touches the pan.

16. Carefully slide it onto plate, cooked side down.

17. Wipe the pan out with a piece of oiled paper towel.

18. With your hand under the plate, lay the frying pan over the frittata.

19. Flip the plate and pan together to transfer the uncooked side of frittata back into the frying pan.

20. Cook 1 to 2 minutes until set.

21. Slip the frittata onto a serving platter and serve in wedges with a crisp salad.

Chicken & Noodles in Coconut Lime Broth

Prepartion time

20 minutes

Ingredients

- 2 teaspoons canola oil

- ½ onion, sliced thin
- 1 clove garlic, sliced thin
- 3-inch piece ginger, peeled and cut into slices
- ¼ teaspoon red pepper flakes, or to taste
- 4 cups chicken broth
- 2 cups coconut milk
- 2 teaspoons lime zest
- 2 teaspoons fish sauce
- ½ pound shiitake mushrooms, sliced (about 2 cups)
- 6 ounces flat rice noodles
- 10 ounces skinless, boneless chicken breast, sliced into thin strips

- ½ cup loosely packed baby spinach or roughly chopped spinach

- ¼ cup fresh lime juice

- 2 tablespoons cilantro leaves, roughly chopped

- 2 stalks scallions, white and light green parts only, sliced

- ½ jalapeño, sliced (optional)

Instructions

1. Heat oil in a medium stockpot over medium-high heat.

2. Cook onions, garlic, ginger, and red pepper flakes just until the onions turn translucent, about 4 minutes.

3. Add the chicken broth, milk, lime zest, and fish sauce.

4. Bring to a boil. Lower to a simmer and add the sliced mushrooms, cook for 5 minutes.

5. Season to taste.

6. Meanwhile, soak and drain the rice noodles according to package instructions.

7. Bring the soup back up to a boil, and add the sliced chicken.

8. Cook until the chicken is no longer pink, about 5 minutes.

9. Stir in the spinach and cook for 2 minutes.

10. Turn off the heat and stir in the lime juice, cilantro leaves, and scallions.

11. Divide the rice noodles between 4 bowls.

12. Pour the hot broth over the noodles.

13. Serve with jalapeño slices, if using.

Kale and Wild Rice Casserole

Prepartion time

1 hour 35 minutes

Ingredients

- 2 large bunches kale, leaves removed from ribs and torn

- 1 cup water

- 4 tablespoons olive oil

- 1 pound cremini mushrooms, sliced

- 1 tablespoon butter

- 2 cloves garlic, minced or grated

- 2 tablespoons fresh thyme, chopped

- ¼ teaspoon nutmeg

- ¼ teaspoon salt, plus more for seasoning

- ½ teaspoon pepper, plus more for seasoning

- 4 tablespoons flour

- 1 cup pasteurized whole milk

- 1 cup chicken or vegetable broth

- ¼ cup coconut milk

- 4 cups cooked wild rice

- 1½ cups grated pasteurized Gruyére cheese

- 2 large sweet onions, sliced into thin rings

Instructions

1. Thoroughly rinse fresh produce under warm running water for 20 seconds. Scrub to remove excess dirt.

2. Preheat oven to 375 degrees. Grease a 2- or 3-quart casserole dish.

3. Heat a very large skillet over medium-high heat.

4. Add kale and water, cover, and cook, stirring occasionally, until kale wilts, 10 to 15 minutes.

5. Once kale is wilted and water is absorbed, remove skillet from heat and use tongs to remove kale to a plate. Set aside.

6. Using tongs, wipe skillet clean with paper towels.

7. Return skillet to medium heat and add 2 tablespoons olive oil.

8. Add mushrooms in a single layer.

9. Cook for 2 minutes without stirring.

10. When bottoms are caramelized, use tongs to turn mushrooms once and season with ¼ teaspoon salt and ½ teaspoon pepper.

11. Continue cooking without stirring for about 5 minutes.

12. Add butter to skillet and cook until it begins to brown.

13. Reduce heat to low and add garlic, thyme, and nutmeg.

14. Cook for about 10 seconds.

15. Add cooked kale and toss to combine.

16. Sprinkle flour over kale mixture and cook for 1 minute.

17. Add whole milk and broth and, stirring, bring to a boil.

18. Reduce heat and cook until thick, 2 to 3 minutes.

19. Add cream and stir to combine.

20. Remove from heat and stir in rice. Pour mixture into prepared dish.

21. Using tongs, wipe skillet clean with paper towels.

22. Add remaining 2 tablespoons olive oil and heat over medium-high.

23. Add onions and salt and pepper to taste.

24. Cook, stirring constantly, until onions begin to soften, about 5 minutes.

25. Continue cooking until onions are golden brown, about 20 minutes.

26. Sprinkle half of the cheese over the casserole, then spread onions in an even layer.

27. Top with remaining cheese.

28. Bake until cheese is melted and onions are crispy, 20 to 25 minutes.

29. Casserole should register 145 degrees Fahrenheit or higher using an instant-read thermometer in the middle of the dish.

Baked Mac & Cheese

Prepartion time

55 minutes

ingredients

- 1/2 cup Cashews raw (soaked for at least 2-3 hours to aid in digestion)

- 16 ounces Brown rice macaroni

- 2 pieces Whole grain or gluten free toast

- 1 cup Filtered water

- 1 cup Unsweetened original almond milk

- 2 tbsp Apple cider vinegar

- 1 tbsp Olive oil
- 1/3 cup Nutritional yeast
- 1 tsp Garlic powder
- 1 tsp Onion powder
- 1 tsp Chili powder
- 1 tsp Salt
- 1/4 tsp Turmeric
- 1/4 tsp Cayenne pepper
- 1/4 tsp Mustard seed

Instructions

1. Place cashews in a bowl and cover with water to let soak for 2-3 hours.

2. Once cashews are done soaking, boil water and cook pasta according to package. You can now also preheat the oven to 350 degrees.

3. While pasta is cooking and the oven is warming up, toast bread and place both pieces in the blender.

4. Blend to form breadcrumb topping, then pour breadcrumbs into a separate bowl or container and set aside.

5. Clean out the blender for use in the next step.

6. Drain and rinse soaked cashews and pour into blender.

7. Add water, almond milk, apple cider vinegar, olive oil, nutritional yeast and all remaining spices.

8. Blend until all ingredients are combined.

9. Once pasta is cooked and strained, place it back into its original pot with the heat turned off.

10. Then pour in the sauce and stir until all pasta is covered.

11. Now pour pasta into your baking dish and make sure it is spread out evenly.

12. Cover the pasta with breadcrumbs (you may have extra depending on the size of bread you used).

13. Place baking dish into the oven uncovered for 20-25 minutes.

14. While the mac & cheese is baking, cook your vegetable of choice to have with the meal.

15. Once done cooking, let the mac & cheese sit for about 5-10 minutes to cool.

16. Then be transported back to your childhood days and enjoy!

Fall Harvest Salad

Prepartion time

1 hour 30 minutes

Ingredients

- 1½ cups chopped butternut or kabocha squash, cut into ½-inch pieces

- 1½ cups chopped carrot, cut into ½-inch pieces

- 1½ cups chopped sweet potato, cut into ½-inch pieces
- 3 tablespoons plus 1 teaspoon olive oil
- 2 teaspoons fresh thyme leaves
- Salt
- 2 medium shallots, peeled, halved, and sliced
- 2 tablespoons lemon juice
- Pepper
- ½ cup toasted, hulled pumpkin seeds
- 2 cups cooked quinoa

Instructions

1. Thoroughly rinse fresh produce under warm running water for 20 seconds.

2. Scrub to remove excess dirt.

3. Preheat oven to 400 degrees. Line a baking sheet with parchment paper.

4. Toss squash, carrot, and sweet potato with 1 teaspoon olive oil, thyme, and a generous pinch of salt.

5. Spread in a single layer on the prepared baking sheet.

6. Bake for 30 minutes, then turn the vegetables and add shallots to the sheet.

7. Bake for an additional 15 minutes.

8. While vegetables are cooking, whisk together remaining 3 tablespoons olive oil, lemon juice, and salt and pepper to taste in a large bowl.

9. Stir in pumpkin seeds and cooked quinoa.

10. When vegetables are tender, let cool slightly, then add to quinoa mixture and stir to combine.

Strawberry Jello Poke Cake

Prepartion time

45 minutes

INGREDIENTS

- 1 16 ounce box angel food cake mix

- 1 3 ounce box strawberry Jello

- 1 cup boiling water

- 1/2 cup cold water

- 2 3.3 ounce boxes white chocolate instant pudding

- 1 1/2 cup milk

- 1 12 ounce container frozen whipped topping, thawed

- 1 pound strawberries

- 1 pint blueberries

INSTRUCTIONS

1. Preheat oven to 350ºF. Do not grease 9-inch by 13-inch pan.

2. Cool completely, at least 1 hour.

3. Using a fork, pierce cake in rows about 1/2-inch apart.

4. When the fork becomes sticky, dip tines in water to clean (typically at the end of each row).

5. Mix angel food cake mix according to package instructions (the one I used only required water).

6. Pour into ungreased pan and bake until firm to the touch, about 30 minutes.

7. If the center still jiggles, bake it 5 minutes longer.

8. Pour Jello into a medium bowl and whisk in boiling water.

9. When Jello is dissolved, stir in cold water.

10. Drizzle over the entire surface of cake.

11. Cover and refrigerate at least 3 hours or overnight.

12. In a large bowl, or in a standing mixer fit with the whisk attachment, combine pudding and milk until well blended.

13. Gently fold in whipped topping.

Chipotle Tomatillo Green-Chili Salsa

Prepartion time

35 minutes

Ingredients

- 2 pounds tomatillos halved
- 3 vine tomatoes halved
- 2 jalapenos deseeded

- 1 red onion cut into wedges
- 4 cloves garlic
- 1 teaspoon kosher salt
- 1/2 teaspoon coarse ground black pepper
- 2 teaspoon cumin
- 1 teaspoon dried oregano
- 2 tablespoons lemon juice
- 2 tablespoons lime juice
- 1/4 cup fresh cilantro

Instructions

1. Preheat your oven to 450 degrees and add the tomatillos, tomato, jalapeñõ and red onion to a

baking sheet and roast for 25-30 minutes until they all start to char.

2. Add the roasted vegetables along with the rest of the ingredients to a large food processor or a blender with a vent (the steam will need an escape) and pulse until slightly chunky, about 10-15 seconds.

Cheesy Spinach Artichoke Dip

Prepartion time

35 minutes

INGREDIENTS

- 8 ounces cream cheese softened

- 1/4 cup mayonnaise
- 1/2 cup grated Parmesan cheese
- 1 clove garlic peeled and minced
- 1/2 teaspoon dried basil
- 1/4 teaspoon salt
- 1/4 teaspoon black pepper
- 14 ounces artichoke hearts drained and chopped
- 10 ounces frozen chopped spinach thawed and drained
- Shredded mozzarella cheese

INSTRUCTIONS

1. Preheat oven to 350 degrees F.

2. Lightly grease a small baking dish.

3. In a medium bowl, mix together cream cheese, mayonnaise, Parmesan cheese, garlic, basil, salt, and pepper.

4. Gently stir in artichoke hearts and spinach.

5. Transfer the mixture to the prepared baking dish.

6. Top with mozzarella cheese.

7. Bake in the preheated oven 25 minutes, until bubbly and lightly browned.

Chai Poh Neng

Prepartion time

18 minutes

INGREDIENTS

- 100 gr sweet chai poh (preserved turnip) You may need less if yours is salty

- 50 gr ground/minced pork + 1 tsp dark soy sauce + 1 tsp brown sugar + 1/2 tsp corn starch optional

- 4 large eggs separate

- 3 Tbsp cooking oil divided

- 1 stalk green onion thinly sliced

- 1/4 tsp sugar if you use salty chai poh

INSTRUCTIONS

Prepare the chai poh:

1. Place the chai poh in a mixing bowl.

2. Cover with clean water and let it soak for about 3 minutes.

3. Drain off the water completely and squeeze out the water as much as you can.

4. Set aside.

5. If using pork, mix the pork with dark soy sauce, sugar, and corn starch.

6. Set aside

7. Roughly chop the chai poh into smaller pieces.

8. You can chop it really fine too if you want to

Prepare the eggs:

1. Separate the yolks from the white.

2. Beat the yolks briefly with a fork or chopsticks and then whisk the white until frothy and pale using a whisk.

3. Then gently fold in the yolks into the white

Cooking:

1. Preheat a large non-stick pan, about 8-10 inch wide.

2. Add 1 Tbsp cooking oil.

3. Stir fry the ground pork and breaking it up with the spatula.

4. Cook until they turn color, about 1 minute.

5. Add chai poh until fragrant and dry, about 10 minutes or so.

6. Add sugar if you use salty chai poh.

7. Have a taste and add more sugar as needed.

8. Dish out the chai poh and pork mixture and set aside

9. Wipe the pan clean if necessary.

10. Bring it back to hot again. It's important that the pan is hot so your omelet won't be greasy.

11. Add another 1 Tbsp cooking oil.

12. Pour in half of the beaten egg and swirl the pan to cover the base of the pan.

13. Use a rubber spatula to push the edge of the omelet to let the runny batter flow in.

14. Repeat as needed to let the runny batter cooks

15. When the egg started to set at the edge but still a bit "wet" in the middle, add half of the chai poh you stir-fried earlier.

16. Sprinkle half of the chopped green onion.

17. Cook until the middle started to set, about 2 minutes and then gently but quickly flip the omelet over to let it cook for another 1 minute or less.

18. Dish out.

19. Bring the pan back to hot again and repeat with another half of the egg and chai poh

Printed in Dunstable, United Kingdom